Pelvic Floor

Simple Poses for Healing Your Body

(An Integrated Program of Pelvic Floor Exercise to Support Overall Pelvic Floor Health)

William Riding

Published By **Ryan Princeton**

William Riding

*Pelvic Floor: Simple Poses for Healing Your Body
(An Integrated Program of Pelvic Floor Exercise to
Support Overall Pelvic Floor Health)*

ISBN   978-1-7750277-2-0

Legal & Disclaimer

The information contained in this book is not designed to replace or take the place of any form of medicine or professional medical advice. The information in this book has been provided for educational & entertainment purposes only.

The information contained in this book has been compiled from sources deemed reliable, and it is accurate to the best of the Author's knowledge; however, the Author cannot guarantee its accuracy and validity and cannot be held liable for any errors or omissions. Changes are periodically made to this book. You must consult your doctor or get professional medical advice before using any of the suggested remedies, techniques, or information in this book.

Table Of Contents

Chapter 1: Connecting to Your Pelvic Floor

05

We are unable to maintain our relationship with

the body is going to transform

spiritual y homeless. Without

An anchor that we can float

unintentionally, battered by

Life's waves and winds.

E A S T E R N B O D Y , W E S T E R N M I N D

06

Be aware of the pelvic floor.

Make sure you are aware of the pelvic floor.

....Did you find it? Are you able to picture the thing? Do you know how to activate it?

What do you know about the intimate area of your body which, over the years has been cloaked by a myriad of cultural stereotypes and religious taboos?

Do we have lost contact to our pelvic floor?

The saying, "If you don't use it, you lose it," can be applied for human biology. The frontal cortex in the brain, there is a distinctive part of the brain that is commonly referred to as the homonculus. It is basically is a representation of the whole body stored in the brain. It is true that there are many maps or homunculi in the brain, two that stand out are the sensory (your brain's interpretations of what you experience) as well as the motor (your brain's controlling of movements throughout your body).

Organs which require greater attention by the brain or, more "brain power" so to put it, have more space in the world map. If, for instance, you're right-handed and have a right hand, the portion of your brain that regulates the motor part of the right hand is more extensive than your left hand since you utilize it for more. For another instance, those who use Braille (often achieved using your index finger) have larger brain regions in the brain which are sensitive to a stimulation with your index finger.

07

It is also possible to think of the brain's map as a sort of filing cabinet in which

3

the folders are organized on each particular body part. If you don't utilize a specific body part, the information inside the brain's area becomes less and less. When less brain power and focus is focused on specific parts of your body, the body tends to go with the flow of effectiveness and makes use of this energy to spend it organizing and managing bigger files that are in the file cabinet, instead of the ones that aren't receiving much attention. It can result in physical and mental dissociation from areas of our bodies.

The dissociation of the pelvic floor may be referred to by many different names. Below are some you've heard (or perhaps even felt yourself):

-Pelvic Organ Prolapse (the descent of pelvic organs to the vagina, or sometimes the vagina)

Incontinence (urine leakage)

Dyspareunia (pain of sexual activity)

Bowel and Bladder Dysfunction

Pelvic Pain/ Low Back Pain

You can see that the loss of our connection to our pelvic floor may not be very desirable. Although many of the issues with pelvic floor can be considered to be normal, they're not typical.

08

Common Normal!

Here are a few facts that have been compiled by the National Institute of Health (NIH) in order to prove that separation from pelvic floor, as well as the dysfunctions that result can be a major cause of illness in the world:

There are more than 25 million Americans have urinary incontinence or leakage. However, many don't seek the treatment.

Research indicates that as high as 50 percent of women who experienced vaginal birth are likely to have pelvic organ prolapse at some point in their life time.

One in seven American women between the ages of 18 and 50 suffers from pelvic pain that lasts at least 3 months.

Because of the taboos and prejudices which are prevalent in our society many people haven't been able to discuss the issues "down there" and have been forced to live by silence and in solitude.

Instead of seeking assistance from family members and medical professionals, patients accept the falsehood that there is no one who could relate to their symptoms/pain and that they're broken and their body is betraying them. The self-deflection that is harmful to the body is untrue.

09

If nobody has ever told you how incredible and strong and enduring your body can be I'm the person to proclaim your praises from the top of my head and let everyone hear about it!

Your body is not broken; you're whole!

Your body's for your benefit, not for!

It is possible to heal!

Make your voice Heard!

If you or your relative is struggling with one of the pelvic floor issues that are listed above, you need to know that you're not alone and you're not in a state of distress, and these problems do not have to play a role in the story of your life. There's an option! There is a solution!

First next step is to reconnect to your pelvic floor.

The great thing is that our brains are extremely flexible, which means it is easily changeable. The great thing about neuroplasticity is that even if we do not like the dimensions of the "Pelvic Floor" folder in the file cabinet of the brain, we are able to alter it! Through increasing our understanding and awareness of our pelvic floor and knowing how to work on activating and reintegrating these muscles with the overall functions of our bodies and mind, we are able to address dysfunctions that result due to pelvic floor dissociation, and change the way we think about health!

10

Clean off the small "Pelvic Floor" file that is tucked away on the bottom of your cabinet.

Uncover the cover on the front.

The time has come to get back in touch to the pelvic floor!

11

Make sure you are aware of the pelvic floor.

Chapter 2: Know Thyself and Thy Pelvic Floor

12

Being aware of yourself is the

The beginning of all wisdom

A R I S T O T L E

13

Be aware of the pelvic floor.

Most of the time, it's an inadequacy of understanding of the pelvic floor which can cause problems. In contrast to other areas of our body, we rarely feel or see the floor of our pelvis often (but should you choose to then, good for you!). Our pelvic floors tend to be "out of sight, out of mind" which is the middle child of our body, as they say. There are a lot of stigmas about what could be wrong "down there" have also caused the pelvic floor to end up being overlooked by the general population as well as the medical profession.

All that has changed today! Nobody puts your

Pelvic floor on the side!

We can begin by re-acquainting ourselves with the pelvic floor, its position, shape, and purpose.

What's the pelvic floor?

The floor of your pelvis is an improvised hammock made comprised of three layers of individual muscles. The first begins at the pubic bone (the bone structure that lies about six inches beneath the belly button) and then travel up towards your Coccyx (your tailbone) and wrap all the way to the left and right ischial tubes (your the sitz bones). The muscles visually create the base of your pelvic bowl.

14

The muscles are wrapped around the openings in the undercarriage. If you are a female at birth or trans-women those openings comprise the vagina, the urethra and the anus. In the case of males assigned at birth, and trans-men those openings comprise the urethra as well as the anus.

The pelvic floor is extremely bloody (large blood vessels).

supply) as well as vastly insularized (a large number of nerves). The

The main nerve is in charge of providing pelvic

the muscles of the floor. Their "spark" is the pudendal nerve. It is the

The nerve's path is a tangled one in its course through

the pelvic bowl, allowing it that reaches all muscles for which it is accountable

the innervating look quite similar to

the transportation infrastructure in Pittsburgh. Whether

If you're traveling through the city or on an afternoon off on Sunday off

move through the pelvic floor. Your GPS will most likely

Most likely to quit, slap out, or wave an white flag. Holy on

and off-roads! (All that praise and appreciation for Pittsburgh and off ramps it's among my top cities! However, can I suggest grids?) What is my pelvic floor supposed to accomplish?

The pelvic floor plays a role for 5 S's. 1. Support

The pelvic floor muscles create the bowl, which protects and supports the abdominal organs like the uterus, bladder and the rectum. Together with the connective tissues of the abdominal cavity and pelvic floor, it plays crucial roles in ensuring that the organs remain where they're meant to be in your body.

15

2. Sphincteric Aid

The muscles of the pelvic floor are wrapped around the openings at the the bowl of the pelvis to assist in closing the rectum and bladder. Also, they aid in keeping Feces, urine, and gas in your body until you're ready to release it. A must-have for allaspiring socialites! If nature is calling to you, the muscles of your pelvic floor relax to permit easy passage to eliminate waste from the body.

*Clinical Note: Studies show that anywhere from 60 to 80 percent of those suffering from pressure urinary incontinence (urine leakage due to pressure for example, sneezing, laughter, or a cough) are able to be ameliorated or eliminated through the pelvic floor muscles. I want to thank my colleagues Pelvic Health Physical Therapists You truly are world changers!

3. Sexual Satisfaction

This is the time to pay attention! A healthy and strong pelvic floor muscles assist in enhancing the tone of the vaginal walls, essential to increase sexual consciousness. For males, the pelvic floor assists in achieving and maintain the desire for an sexual errection. The muscles of the pelvic floor ease to permit painless perforation (this is the case with intercourses with tampons, toys and other strange objects that my ER nursing colleagues need to remove surgically from their patients before telling me their horror stories during our meals.)

16

4. Stability

The pelvic floor forms an integral part of the "deep core" and plays crucially to stabilize the spinal column. This helps avoid pain and discomfort higher up and lower down in the kinetic chain (joints between the two levels).

*Clinical note If you're experiencing lower back or the sacroiliac (SI) discomfort it is likely that there's a likelihood that your pelvic floor requires reminding of the job purpose.

5. Sump Pump

The muscles of the pelvic floor assist in lymphatic drainage as well as the circulation of blood vessels and venus. Similar to the calf muscles that are located in your legs, which act like pumps that move lymph and blood back toward your heart, your pelvic floor also performs exactly the same process. When the sump pump in our bodies aren't functioning well, constriction and swelling develop.

.....AND additionally the posture, breathing and breath!

The two subjects are huge! In fact, they are so significant that they should be the title of their own book! The subject will be covered further in the coming pages. It's a great way to finish a story!

This is a tip Diaphragm and pelvic floor is the most favored of friends. Ride-or-dies. BFFS 4eva. Together, they bring breath into and out from your body. Where the breath moves and your attention is focused, it follows!

The reason is that breath and posture are closely linked too!

17

Also, I'm sure that you and your pelvic floor could reconnect and catch up, enjoy drinks together and begin to revive the relationship! The pelvic floor provides you with many blessings maybe this is the an appropriate time to show it the respect and love it is due!

Read on to find out how your pelvic floor is in sync with your body, and also is a key component in the functioning of the core!

18

Make sure you are aware of the pelvic floor.

Chapter 3: The "Core" of the Matter 19

Yoga poses that you should do not want to be doing

Most likely is the one that you'll require the

most.

THELITTLEREDBOOKOF

YOGAWISDOM

20

I could feel the voice of my yoga instructor in my head while I wrote out the line. It's true, but isn't it?

If you gravitate towards fast-paced, single-breath-to-single-movement power yoga and avoid the stillness and deep connective tissue mobilization of yin yoga like the plague...there is a good chance yin is what your body is craving.

If you're anything like me, and feel a bit numb in your stomach every time you feel that your class may be entering the "core phase" of the training, then it's the perfect indication that your body needs care and attention.

Do not get me wrong, I'm a huge fan of the core! Every movement of the body gets better when the muscles are strong and prepared for motion. It is essential to strengthen our core! After years of pounding my abs to submission using sitting-ups and crunches, as well as trying to figure out what was wrong with my breathing and posture patterns were strained and why my six-pack didn't seem to be able to come into my life, the idea that I was doing "core work" brings back doubts about my fitness and inadequacy.

It was the truth that I was never able to comprehend what was the fundamental. In the absence of a complete knowledge of its core my efforts to understand and build it failed.

We'll get closer to our "core" of the matter! Let's discuss the "core!

21

There was a belief that the core consisted only of the abdominal muscles that were superficial, also known as the muscles that comprised the 6-pack. Further research has revealed that the deep core actually a set of muscles that cooperate and provide support to the spine as well as the pelvis. They create the supportive and safe "canister" that wraps around your midsection, supporting the pelvis and spine as well as control the pressure gradients within the human body (i.e. to ensure that you don't break your abdominal muscles whenever you cough, laugh or sneeze. Hernias aren't easy to deal with).

If we are talking about the muscles which make up the core of your body there are four primary participants that comprise the front, back sides, the top as well as the bottom canister for the core. Let's look into the roles of each of these players!

1. Diaphragm (The Lid of the Canister) The diaphragm (also known as the Lid of the Canister) is shapely sheet of skeletal muscles which divides your heart and lung lungs located in your thoracic cavity, and the organs of the abdomen. cavity. It relaxes and contracts in sync by breathing to permit air to enter and out of your body.

Inhaling, your lung expands and is filled with air. The diaphragm relaxes and decreases in order to let air be drawn into your body.

Inhalation is a breath of exhalation. lung's lungs relax, and the diaphragm contracts eccentrically (energetically extends) when it returns to its normal position permitting air to escape from the body.

22

The diaphragm is in sync to your breath, and also in sync with the next component of our central system.

2. The Pelvic Floor (The Floor of the Canister) The diaphragm breathing, and the pelvic floor are your 3 greatest friends you could be blessed to They are all connected and function throughout the body. comprise three

In addition to making phone calls, they are adorned with friendship bracelets that match to make sure they don't leave the bathroom by themselves.

A well-functioning and healthy core as your diaphragm expands when you inhale and exhale, your pelvic floor lengthens and expands so that air has the space it needs to move around the body.

When you exhale, your diaphragm relaxes, returning to its normal position and your pelvic floor also follows by contracting, and then gradually lifting upwards toward the top of your head.

*Clinical Notification: This sync connection between the diaphragm breath, as well as the pelvic floor needs to be maintained during lifting heavy weights or coughing. It is also important to keep it in sync when you are sn and laughing. If connection between these three groups fails to occur, then urine leakage (stress incontinence) as well as other problems with the pelvic area could develop.

3. Transversus Abdominus (Front/Sides of the Canister)The transversus abdominus or TVA abbreviated, comprises one of the largest abdominal muscle that is found in our body. It functions as an inner corset or weight belt. It wraps across the front of the body back towards the spine.

Do you see any powerlifters in the gym, putting their swoles in while sporting a fashionable belt that wraps around their pelvis and back? The belt mimics what happens to the TVA. TVA -

the body's own weight belt.

The TVA can be moved by breathing and breath. (Are you getting the sense that proper breathing is crucial to ensure the muscles are functioning correctly and sync up with the various muscles in your body? You can trust my intuition!).

Inhaling, the TVA is pushed outwards and away from your spine so that the stomach can expand to take up the smallest part of your lung.

After exhaling On exhalation, the TVA is pushed inwards, toward the spine. The belly sinks back towards the spine.

*Clinical note: Training to train the TVA to contract on its own as well as in sync with the core posse vital prior to beginning the traditional core workouts. This will ensure that the lower back is secure and comfortable and that the pressure gradients are assisting the body, not against it.

24

The TVA can be located TVA using your fingertips in the bony projections located at the top of your pelvis. (These bony projections represent the Anterior Superior Iliac Spines (ASIS) in case we need to go into technical. This information is useful when you're preparing for an intense sport like Hangman). For you to be able to feel the TVA activate, lie on your back, with your knees bent, and your feet on the floor. Your fingers should be pressing on the inside of your ASIS to pull your belly button to your spine, and then turn your pelvis toward the top of your head. If you're a Cowboy or woman, consider bringing the buckle of your belt to the hat of your cowboy. Have you felt a muscle spring up in your hands? I'd like to introduce the TVA. Yeehaw!

4. Multifidus (Back of the Canister) The multifidi comprise the short muscles

running along the spine, from the tailbone of your body to your occipital bone at the bottom of the skull. They collaborate with the rest of their family members to help support and safeguard the spine resulting in secure and safe motion patterns.

*Medical Note: If you experience an ongoing low back pain that appears to be a mild pain, it is possible strengthen the muscles. However, the multifidi tend to be overlooked when it comes to training programs, resulting in these muscles being forced to strain themselves to overcome other weakness as well as muscle imbalances within the body (like weakness in the abdominals).

25

The diaphragm, pelvic floor TVA and mutifidus have to be sturdy as individuals They also have to master coordination in order to "play well together." If any of the four players aren't invited to the gathering and the system isn't properly coordinated, it can go badly and unhealthful movements develop that can result in pain and dysfunction. Core muscles are activated the muscles, or activates, to anticipate movements. That means, before you begin the process of lifting your arms up to begin your first session in Sun As, the muscles that make up your core are triggering to anticipate your movements. The anticipation reaction is involuntary...but when your brain isn't equipped to handle this type of motor behavior it will require some retraining of your brain, too! (Refer to Chapter 01 for a conceptual understanding of the best way to modify your brain to be able to perform effective motion patterns! It's brainwashing in the best way!) Once we know the anatomy of our core, the muscles involved in coordination, and the way they work in order to protect and support our bodies, we are able to improve our understanding of how to correctly activate the muscles to strengthen them and use this system of protection in order to stay safe from injuries and live more healthy lives both in and out of the mat!

26

What is the best way to activate the pelvic floor, and connect all the muscles in our system of support to prevent unsafe movement patterns that may result in pain and dysfunction?

Thanks for the question! Stay with me, so that we can continue learning and exploring our incredible human bodies.

27

Make sure you are aware of the pelvic floor.

Chapter 4: How To Find & Activate Your Pelvic Floor

28

May your coffee, pelvic

floors, intuition and self-confidence

Appreciation should remain robust.

U N K N O W N

29

"Engage your pelvic floor" is a call that is frequently taught in yoga classes. However, what exactly does this refer to and how do we achieve that?

In the beginning, you can read a short spark note overview of the pelvic floor (or if you're member of the 1 percent of students who don't utilize spark-notes in high school to be able to pass their English class, then you'll be able to take a look at the entire and unabridged description on the pelvic floor at Chapter 02!). If you're one of the of us who are lazy, check out this article!

The pelvic floor is a body consisting of three distinct layers of muscle that join the pubic bone at the forward part of the pelvis. It connects the coccyx (tailbone) in the back of the pelvis. The pelvis it then spreads to the ischial tubes (sitz bones) to the sides. The pelvic floor plays a role for many important functions throughout the human body.

Remember the 5 S's?? It's Quiz Time!

The resume of the pelvic floor can be summarized like this: 1. The pelvic floor has the responsibility to provide support for all organs of the pelvic bowl. This includes the bladder, rectum and the uterus 2. Spinctering to ensure that gas, urine and feces go out of your body when you provide it with the green signal to do that.

30

3. Stabilizing the pelvis and spinal bones to prevent dysfunctional patterns of movement

4. acting as a sump-pump for pumping lymph and blood into the heart to ensure it isn't weakened by gravity's forces and leak into the lower parts of your body. The process of making sex legend...wait to hear it...dary! (The kind that is respectful and mutually agreed to kind of course!) The pelvic floor is an important player in the area of breathing and posture. These are something that us, as humans of today struggle with a hard at doing correctly. To be fair, it's not entirely our fault.

We're part of the environment we live in After all.

The fact is that our body was designed to move, not sit in a chair for eight hours every day keeping track of the minutes until we are able to go home and head home for a Netflix watch. Are you familiar with the saying "Sitting is the new smoking?" It's true. According to the American College of Occupational and Environmental Medicine Sitting might be the single least understood health risk in the present.

(Unfortunately We'll have to speak about the effects of sitting on our bodies in a different book! It's a spoiler: the message of the story is to move! Start a timer, and then move at least 3-5 minutes every hour. Take care of your body. You are entitled to receive compassion, and especially by yourself.) 31

So, How Do We Activate The Pelvic Floor?

Good question! Keep in mind that the pelvic floor has been linked to breathing and functions in sync with diaphragm. If we are able to breathe deeply and use our diaphragm (a breathing method known as diaphragmatic breathing) then we will be able to effortlessly activate our pelvic floor.

This is a simple way to identify and strengthen the pelvic floor. Check this out!

1. Begin by finding your supportive hero's pose using an bolster or a yoga block. For this position your prop should lie placed between your knees, and then rest on your peritoneum. You should be seated tall, and feeling the upward force of the bone's ridge that runs along the top your skull (the Occipital Ridge) in

order to lengthen your spine while promoting the support you need to maintain your position.

2. Your hands should be placed on your stomach.

3. Breathe in deeply when you take a long breath through your nostrils. Inhale deeply and allow your stomach to expand. Then push out with those palms. As you inhale, imagine the shape of a balloon that is resting inside your pelvic and stomach which you inflate by inhaling each time. Imagine your area of your pelvis expanding when the ballon press against it. If you're a visual person think that the pelvic floor is blossoming and expanding as the lotus flower (or the flower that you are choosing...I'm one of the sunflower people Secret admirers, be aware!).

32

4. The air will dance around the red balloon that is resting inside the pelvic area. Then exhale with pursed lips in the same way as you blow your birthday candles.

(Make an wish! The draft was clearly composed prior to COVID

When blowing out birthday candles didn't endanger grandma's existence). Your hands will sink toward your spine, as air leaves your body. After exhaling, the aim is to experience some gentle lifting of the pelvic floor off the support. In anatomy, the movement from the pelvic floor occurs as a mild squeeze, or a zipping of the orifices at the pelvis' bottom (urethra, rectum and vagina) and an upward movement towards the top of the head. The fun commences. ....

In order to achieve the energetic lifting that the pelvic floor muscle from the bolster, it is necessary to locate an activation signal for the pelvic floor that is effective to your advantage! If you're well-adjusted the pelvic floor, and your body-brain connection is healthy the physical cues that the support is rubbing against your perineum could be the only thing you require. However, if you're in need of additional assistance try some of these visual cues. Select the one you like best! (Parental discretion admonished The authors aren't afraid of speaking about anatomy throughout this book! If you hadn't been paying attention!).

Pelvic Floor Activation Cues:

Imagine closing all the holes at the lower part of your pelvis and then lifting them into your body for 33

Imagine picking one of the blueberries with your anus

Imagine your genital area as straws and imagine you're taking a big slushy drink

Imagine that the pelvic floor acts as an elevator. As you breathe out then the doors will close and the elevator rises until the 3rd floor.

Imagine that your pelvic floor acts as an eddiefish squeezing itself into and then soaring upwards toward the top of the ocean.

OR create your own idea for a cue! I guarantee it, physical therapists who specialize in pelvic health would be thrilled to have more cues for visualization to their toolbox!

Practice Makes Perfect: Become The Master of Your Pelvic Floor

The pelvic floor muscles are activated in anticipation of movement.

So, before you make any movement in your body the pelvic floor and the core system as together, will kick into motion to support your middle section. It means that your pelvic floor needs to be loosening gently and relaxing to the rhythm of your breathing as you anticipate each posture transition.

34

An effective way to prepare the pelvic floor to ensure proper alignment and retrain your mind to focus on the central system is to do the method before every yoga class, while lying on your mat, and creating your mantra/intention for the yoga practice.

Then, the sequence of your pelvic floor by breathing and movements will be automatic and you'll no longer need to use any mental energy behind it.

However, until that day comes Practice, practice, practise!

It's been said that it requires 100,000 hours of training to perfect a skill. Learn to master your pelvic floor, by chipping away at the hours you spend in your yoga mat prior to each yoga class!

35

If you've completed reading this chapter and were thinking,

"Hey! This whole pelvic floor activation thing sounds a lot like engaging mula bandha. or the root lock!,"

You're on the right track!

Keep following me, and we'll examine this issue deeper as we continue our tour through the human body.

Connecting the research of physical therapy to the practice and technique of yoga!

36

Be aware of the pelvic floor.

Chapter 5: Oo La La, Mula Bandha!

37

You should be able to move your weight towards al that

feels supportive. Inspiring.

Expansive. Warm. Frequent

these spaces for as long as it's

Habitual, you will not need

Anything other than. Then you are created.

to feel this feeling of

belonging. Because you

belong.

V I C T O R I A E R I C K S O N

38

When I tell anyone I meet the fact that I'm an Pelvic Health Physical Therapist I often get either of these response:

1. "Oh yeah, pelvic health! So you teach women to do kegels all day? That's it?!" OR

2. "Pelvic Health Therapist?! Wait, are you like a Sex Therapist?!"

Both responses are not 100% accurate and neither are they completely incorrect. One of the responses I receive more frequently during Bumble dates.

It's true that this Pelvic Health Movement has only earned its spot in the spotlight of healthcare only recently. However, it's one which is growing with a dazzling speed with more and more people speaking out and making their voices heard regarding their own personal experiences dealing with the pelvic health issue.

While education and help for pelvic health, which is just beginning to show signs of progress in the western world, recognizing the significance of taking care of the pelvic floor isn't something new.

One could claim that the very first

Health advocates for the pelvic area were early yogis! The first to promote the concept of the kegel were first to establish our yoga exercise!

39

Are you still not sure? Take a look at this passage of the Upanishads (an old Sanskrit text that describes several of the theories of the spiritual practices in yoga):

"By contracting the perineum the downward moving apana vayu is forced to go upward. Yogis call this mula bandha. Press the heel firmly against the rectum and contract forcefully and repeatedly, so that the vital energy rises. There is no doubt that by practicing mula bandha, prana and apana, and nada and bindu, are united, and total perfection is attained."

We'll break it down! What is the issue there?

In traditional yoga, it is believed that there are channels of energy/prana/life-force that flow throughout and energize the body. The main channel of energy flows from the top of the head. It then exits at the bottom of the spine. It is at the the pelvic floor. The central channel is often called the shashumna-nadi. The flow of energy which goes down the downward direction is known as apana-vayu.

To stop the flow this energy apana-vayu and its downward exit of the body, ancient yoga practitioners would use mula bandha a powerful movement of the pelvic floor muscles, which could bring about sphincteric control over the orifices located at the bottom of the pelvis (urethra, vagina, rectum) which would stop the energy flow through the body.

40

The term bandha is a reference to "to bind" or "to lock."

In the yoga tradition there are three main bandhas within the body. There is the fourth bandhas that tie them all:

Mula Bandha (The Root Lock)

Uddiyana Bandha (The Abdominal Lock)

Jalandhara Bhanda (The Throat Lock)

-Maha Bhanda (The Mother of all Bandhas is a mix consisting of Mula, Uddiyana, and Jalandhara Bandhas)

If you are able to engage the mula bandha as well as "lock" the muscles of the pelvic floor (aka those in the pelvic floor) the result is an alteration in the flow of energy in your body. Instead of the apana-vayu energy moving upwards and out of the body lands on the pelvic wall, which is closed then swirls in the lower part of the spine and returns to the top of the head, invigorating the body at the core of who you are. (If you do kundalini yoga it is likely that you're getting goose bumps when you think about that dancing energy in the bottom of your spine that is awakening the serpent kundalini!)

41

My favourite portion of this passage of the Upanishads is the way it explains the ways that ancient yogis employed the sensation of a touch to activate the pelvic muscles of the floor. There's a deep-seated physical reason for them to be practically putting their heels in to show off their tummy!

Muscles react to physical stimulation (i.e. it is possible to draw brainpower in the form of intention, awareness and concentration towards a the muscle group by tapping it using your fingertips or using a proprioceptive signal such as the piece of athletic tape or kinesio-tape on the stomach of your muscles). In the article, yoga yogis use their heel set against the rectum in order to signal the muscles of the pelvic floor to activate to signal the muscles to pull together upwards towards the top of the head. This is producing a lift sensation of the heel of your foot, which you feel. If you experience a feeling of lift-off you're engaged the mule bandha and making sure you are kegel-ing to strengthen the abdominal muscles!

(This is precisely that we covered at the end of Chapter 04! Reread Chapter 04 for a detailed explanation of the best way to prepare the mula bandha (pelvic muscles that contract in the floor/kegel) for a full engagement when you are sitting in your yoga mat! As we've discussed in the method in Chapter 04, we're using an bolster for that sensory cue. You might want to consider using the heel of your feet as a more cost-effective method to achieve the same result (minimalists are encouraged!)).

42

I'd like to also mention that the earliest yoga practitioners were males. People who were aware that taking care of the pelvic floor wasn't solely "women's work." EVERYONE

is a pelvic floor, and deserves just the same amount of attention, respect and consideration like the rest of your body!

Spending the time to connect with your pelvic floor will bring you the advantages of improved the control of your pelvic floor, better urinary and bowel function as well as stronger gastric orgasms (just to mention some!).

When your instructor in yoga instructs you to activate mula Bandha, it is the "root lock," the Kegel, which is the dynamic lifting of abdominal muscles of the pelvic floor .....GO for it! It might be surprising how this tiny instruction can transform your exercise routine!

43

Contrary to the response number 1, which is mentioned at the start in this section, I don't advise women or men to perform kegels every day ALL DAY. Actually, there are many reasons strengthening the pelvic floor may be a contraindication for certain people who suffer from pelvic floor problems.

The pelvic floor is muscle group, as is any other muscle one must be able to contract fully and completely relax to ensure that it is well-maintained and efficient. The pelvic floor can suffer from a variety of issues. result when the muscles of the pelvic floor aren't capable of fully relaxing.

Keep going with us on our way together! There's a lot more exploring to do! The body is an amazing place!

44

Be aware of the pelvic floor.

Chapter 6: Kegels

Alright or All Hype?

45

One who looks out, hopes;

Whoever looks within, wakes up.

C A L R J U N G

46

If we're going to discuss Kegels, we should be sure to show respect for her Kegel queen herself Tatyana Kozhevnikova.

While she's probably not one of the household names (unless you're a follower of the discipline known as "Intimate Weightlifting"), Tatyana is the Guinness World Record holder holding 14 kilograms (30.8 pounds) using the abdominal muscles.

Impressive? Very.

Handy? You bet that she doesn't have to make two trips in order to transport all her food items.

As we have discussed in the preceding chapters, the gradual pulling upwards and downwards of the muscles in the pelvic floor that form the pelvic bowl's floor bowl, is the basis that allows the contraction of the pelvic floor. AKA the Kegel. The pelvic floor is strong and is vital for the performance of a variety of essential functions within the body. For instance:

Be sure that your abdominal organs are in the place the nature designed (preventing the pelvic organ from prolapse)

Ensure that "laughing until you pee" doesn't become a common incident

(though I would like to hope you have the best leak-free happiness and joy all over the globe!)

Insuring that you have a healthy bladder and bowel

The art of making sex more sexual

47

Take note that hanging the coconut or surfboard out of the vagina did do not qualify for it onto the "Vital Functions of the Pelvic Floor List." We salute you Tatyana with all your wacky pelvic floor tricks!

Should We Believe the Hype?

In the last few years Kegels have received lots of buzz. If you've had a baby or childbirth, then you've probably had a medical professional hurriedly leaving the exam room and putting their hand on the shoulder of their patient an enthralling, quick remark of

"Remember to do your kegels, dear!"

*Clinical Notification: In a thoroughly documented and cited study concerning the effectiveness of kegels using only verbal instructions (Bump 1991) researchers instructed 47 women to properly perform a the kegel.

Of the 47 people who participated...

60% of patients had made effective efforts while 40% of those not doing the right thing. 25 percent of the patients who did it totally wrong, were engaging in practices which increased the frequency of urinary incontinence (instead of delaying it) 48

It is safe to say that simply instructing people to do the kegels will not be aiding, and could cause more harm than positive. Understanding WHAT

The pelvic floor, where it's located the reason why it's so crucial, how to correctly connect it and how to provide it with some love to ensure it is able to perform the job it was intended to. .....THAT is pelvic floor education everyone needs! (I'm slowing stepping down from my ranting here, but take a moment to go through Chapter 04 to see the pelvic floor's tyraid going on all cylinders!) How did kegels come to begin and do they actually work good as they're advertised to be? Are kegels that simple one of the "magic pill" for all problems with the pelvic floor?

In The Beginning: Dr. Arnold Kegel Pelvic Health Hero OR Kegel-Craze Hype-Man?

The late 1940s saw Gynecologist Arnold Kegel, made an crucial observation when working with his female patients suffering from the problem of urinary incontinence post-childbirth. Kegel concluded that strengthening the muscle pubococcygeal (located at the bottom of three

Pelvic floor layers) The clients of his had less leakage and an improvement in sexual health.

49

In order to expand his study and determine the strength of pelvic floor muscles that are of interest He invented a device that could measure the strength of contractions that are voluntary to the pelvic floor. He named"the perineometer.. The results of his research were published in 1948.

He also defended the radical concept that urinary incontinence could be managed with surgical intervention. Simply by retraining and strengthening your pelvic floor muscles the doctor argued that fewer people required to undergo surgery under the knife in order to get the relief they need from leakage!

Kegels are "curing" pelvic health dysfunctions since the 1940s when they first came out, how come so many women are having pelvic pain, urinary pelvic organ prolapse as well as erectile dysfunction as well as bowel and bladder issues?

It is true that there are many reasons. First, the reason that we discussed earlier in the chapter.

The majority of people aren't getting the proper knowledge and instruction to execute Kegels in a correct manner. This is in addition to the fact that many of us feel completely disconnected from the pelvic floor and have a diminished awareness of what is "down below," and are unsure of about how to activate these smaller-known areas of our complex and wonderful bodies, and it's the perfect sense that a verbal guideline about how to do the kegel, along with reminders each month to "keep up the good work," simply isn't going be enough.

50

The shameless promotion of Pelvic Health Physical Therapy here!

Incorporating a Pelvic Health PT (PHPT) in your group can help a lot! They are not just equipped to guide you through ways to improve your health and wellbeing on your pelvic floor but they also conduct an extensive assessment of your pelvis to determine the need for kegels to you.

However, they do not provide the perfect solution to solve all our problems with pelvic health! Actually the majority of cases, they are a no-no and are completely unsuitable! Find out more about essential muscle knowledge and their role in Kegels!

Muscle Truths

Be aware the pelvic floor made up of MUSCLES which were designed to perform certain tasks similar to all other muscles in the body.

So, here are some essential muscle truths facts applicable to all muscles. These are the ones we need to remember when we make sure that the pelvic floor muscles remain healthy and performing their job effectively.

Muscle Truth #1: All Muscles Must Be Able to Fully Relax and Fully Contract

Check out your Bicep. The most well-known uses of the bicep stretching (bending) the elbow as well as controlling the rate of extension of your elbow.

The elbow's flexion is a central phase of motion so the bicep's length is reducing and producing the force.

51

Extending the elbow can be described as the eccentric motion phase The bicep's length extends while creating force.

For the greatest power to be produced through a muscle is to function, it must be able to demonstrate all the range of motion, including fully concentric and eccentric phase.

Imagine having the arm in a cast, with your elbow bent at 90 degrees for three months (let's suppose that ninjas have some connection with the fact that you're being cast because any good story about injury should include a ninja-like heroics!). If the casting is taken off the bicep won't extend fully since it was placed with a shorter position for a long period. Your bicep's strength is also diminished because it will no longer be able to produce forces throughout its whole movement. If you visit Physical Therapy, the primary thing that the PT will assist with is gaining that complete range of motion.

You will then focus on re-strengthening your muscles!

Similar analogies apply to the gluteal floor muscles!

If the muscles of your pelvic floor have been shortened that isn't able to relax fully and lengthen, they'll become fragile.

A muscle that is shortening can be weak muscles! (It's an intriguing notion to consider if were told your hip flexors are tight. Are you actually suffering from hip flexors that are tight or are you suffering from weak hip flexors after working for hours?

Do you work for a long time with your muscle confined to a contracted posture (hip extension)? You have a high probability that you should strengthen the hip flexors rather than demanding an hour of hip flexor stretching during the Yin Yoga class!

It's fun to study physiology!)

52

Muscle Truth #2: Hypotonic and Hypertonic Muscles MUST Be Addressed CORRECTLY

If a muscle is excessively active (or constantly "turned on") and at a reduced position, we are able to impress acquaintances at parties making use of the word "HYPERTONIC" to define the state of our muscles. Hyperis a greek word, which means "excess." Tonic is a greek word which means "excess."

"tone." Hypertonic is a term used to describe excessive muscle tone. That's it!

(Everything originates from the Greeks. If you aren't convinced I will provide you a full hour of talk about how every major achievement in the world is directly inspired by the Greeks until you're exhausted to a point.)

The hypertonic muscle, or the group of muscles must be taught to relax in order that it can produce force effectively. If your bicep muscle is hypertonic it isn't the first thing you should take an oversized dumbbell of 50 pounds and begin pounding through repetitions. This would set you to suffer from discomfort and disfunction. This is also true of the thigh and pelvic floors. If muscles are being overly "turned on," we do not want to force them off with Kegels. Instead, we should train them to lower and relax muscles to ensure that they can completely lengthen and extend and ensure the full range of motion as well as efficient performance.

If you suffer from high-grade pelvic floor, Kegels should not be your friends. They may allow for you to join them at the table at lunch or be observed at the entrance However, they're not your friends, and they are not keeping your best interests at heart. #Frenemy.

53

Hypotonic muscles (decreased muscles) require training to "turn on" appropriately. The muscles must be re-trained, and taught how to work.

A greater awareness for the muscles in question will increase the connection between brain and body, and will allow the muscles to "wake up" and be conscious of their role is within the body. (The the spirit animal for muscles when they are in this state is the legendary sloth. They're cute however you don't wish to emulate their laid-back, slothful and relaxed lifestyle.) If you're suffering from hypotonic bicep you need to make that muscle stronger. Start with a gentle 5#

dumbbells, and begin pumping with reps. You can then gradually add weight until the muscle is prepared to carry loads. If your bicep muscle has trouble remembering it's supposed to do and to begin a contraction then it is possible that a PT could hook the Bicep to an electric stimulation to provide extra electrical stimulation so that it will get more powerful.

This is also true of the floor of your pelvis. When your pelvic floor has been "turned off"if the brain-body link has been cut off due to a absence of awareness related to the area of our bodies and if there's an injury or trauma to the area which is causing your body to not know how to use and coordinate these muscles properly and properly then kegels might be part of your health care plan for pelvic issues. Similar to the bicep analogy stimulation is also a way for "wake up" the pelvic floor muscles. It sounds alarming but it's a very useful device!

54

If your pelvic floor is getting stronger, you are able to boost your weight load by increasing your kegel repetitions or by using smaller internal weights. If lifting chandeliers and surfboards by using your pelvic floor one of your goals then go for it! There is a chance that you will be your next Intimate Weightlifting Champion and bring home the gold medal as part of Team USA! As a Pelvic Health PT, I have found that having the ability to control your pelvic floor muscles during a full spectrum of functional, everyday activities (squats, lifting, double unders in crossfit, rooting to rise into Warrior 1) is way more functionally beneficial than suspending interesting inanimate objects from your undercarriage....but, you do you!

Don't let me ruin your Olympic goals!

How can we be sure our pelvic floors are fully extending and contracting in order to generate maximum strength and perform their task when we sweat it out on yoga mats? Connecting our pelvic floor contractions/kegels/mula bandha with our diaphragmatic breathing is KEY! The breath acts as the ignition switch that triggers the pelvic floor to go into high gear, and to coordinate to the rest of our core system!

Switch on the key, and your heart pumping!

Inhale deeply take a moment to let your breath stretch your belly and move into your pelvic bowl. This will let the pelvic floor grow and blossom as an octopus. If you're looking for a healthy pelvic floor and a healthy core in training, getting your pelvic floor to be fully relaxed is essential!

55

These are yoga postures that can help pelvic floor muscles stretch and relax while you take the diaphragmatic breath

Happy Baby Pose

Child's Pose

Malasana Squat

Goddess Squat

Downward Facing Dog

What do these poses share in the same? They all aid in opening up the lower part of the pelvis, and lengthen your muscle of pelvic floor.

If you exhale visualize or use a visual cue to press and raise the pelvic floor muscles. (Go through Chapter 04 for a complete collection of interesting and fun visualization techniques!). Check to see if you are able to co-ordinate the contraction of your pelvic floor every breath you take in during an exercise routine. Consider a conscious anchor for a more meditative exercise! It will require lots of coordinated brain power as you begin (especially when you're just beginning to re-acquaint yourself with the pelvic floor) However, eventually, the pelvic floor will be able to remember the task it was made to accomplish, will be equipped with the power and flexibility of motion needed to work in its optimal way and will begin to function in a way that isn't necessary to be thinking about it. It's the aim!

56

Read Muscle Truth #3 below to discover how you can

Optimize your kegels for strengthening the pelvic floor

Muscles on and off the mat!

Muscle Truth #3: Muscles Have "Dark Meat" and

"White Meat"

There you are at Thanksgiving Dinner and Uncle Mike is cutting up the turkey. "Do you want white meat or dark meat?," Uncle Mike inquires.

The pelvic floor is the first topic we'll interrupt in this blog to present you with an introductory essay on the anatomy and physiology of turkeys. ....

Thus, turkeys participate in turkey-related behaviors. Turkey's muscles must be able to support these behaviors. Turkeys require the ability to stand for extended times and must also be able to fly for short distances. They require muscle endurance to sustain long walks and the strength to fly in short bursts.

Turkey muscle and human muscle, are made up of a variety of muscles fibers. There are two main types of fibers -

one type of fiber that is suited for endurance activities (slow muscles, twitch fibers Type 1) as well as one type to provide short periods of energy (fast muscles, twitch fibers Type 2.). The science of muscle has discovered a few different fiber types that are not listed, but in our discussion about turkeys we'll stay with these two types of fibers.

57

Slow-twitch (Type 1) muscles are natural and aerobic. This means they use oxygen to generate energy by the triphosphate of adenosine (ATP).

ATP is the most usable form of energy within the body. It's the portion that goes into the machine that pinballs the body, to let all the fun sound and lights going! The Type-1 muscle fibers have a resistance to fatigue which means they're ideal for endurance-based sports (90 minutes of endurance yoga classes or triathlons, marathons in the race to beat the record for plank, etc.). When you look at them, they appear lighter in hue and are, in essence, the

"dark meat" of the"dark meat" in the.

Fast Twitch (Type 2) muscle fibers tend to be anaerobic (not huge consumers of oxygen) for their metabolic functions.

They're faster at wear out and thus are best suitable for short bursts of energy and endurance (power lifting, cranking out sprints, chaturanga pushups swipe right on dating apps or other apps, etc.). In images, these muscles appear to be less luminous hello "white meat."

Every muscle in the body, fast-twitch and slow-twitch muscles are with each other in perfect harmony. According to estimates, half of the muscles in our body belong to Type 1,. 50% are Type 2. (25 25% Type 2a,

25 25% Type 2x, and between 1 to 3 percent Type 2c, to be exact...these diverse types that make up Type two muscle fibres distinguish the minor differences in the way they create ATP and are a fun information to share during parties (and increase the Cool factor).

58

The amount of fiber types is present in each of your muscles can be affected by genetic factors, conditions, and other the effects of age.

Genetics influence the level of nerve stimulation to each muscle fiber. The way nerves work is that they inform muscles of what they should do. They must be in contact with muscles that they are transmitting instructions to. If there are many nerves communicating with Type 1 muscle fibers, these muscle fibers are likely to play a larger role on how your body functions (in this case, sprinting is probably not the best choice for you). It is the same when you have nerves communicating to Type 2 muscles.

Muscle fibers (in this instance you'll notice that sprints tend to be the most prominent within your wheelhouse).

Training-related factors that are specific to your needs can trigger tiny variations (~10 percent) in the muscle fiber's type. It's possible that there could be a smaller percent of types of muscle which change in their structure depending on the demands that are put on the body. The human body is incredibly flexible! If you make the decision to run ultramarathons and begin doing an abundance of endurance exercises the possibility is that your body may transform the Type 2 muscle fibres, that are better suited for quick bursts of speed to Type 1 muscles, that are better suited to endurance. It is similar when you are to train constantly using sprints, or even olympic lifting.

59

Aging is an inevitable process. It happens to everyone. If you're a yoga instructor and you're training your body to adapt to ageing and the end-of-the-world curtain by completing the savasana (corpse posture) after each session of yoga. As the years pass, we lose muscles of the Type 2 variety. BUT

Remember how flexible your body can be? Even as you age there is no reason not to work to build strength. You can be 100

decades old, still pumping up chaturanga push-ups every time you do vinyasa! I have a customer aged 101 who is able to do squats using a weight of 25lbs.

kettlebell ....go to the next level and attempt to prove that the resiliency and adaptability of the human body aren't just one of the greatest things about it? !

Let's not let Uncle Mike in the dark on his Thanksgiving turkey-carving problem. ....

Uncle Mike would like to know whether you prefer white meat and dark meat. The white meat is found inside the breast of the turkey which is where brief bursts of energy are required to assist the turkey travel small distances (more than 2 miles).

fibers). Dark meat can be found within the thighs and legs where endurance is more important for them to be able to run around for hours and pound the ground or do any other thing turkeys spend their day long doing (more Fibers of Type 1.).

60

Then, put your chin to the sky, and look Uncle Mike directly at him without flinching,

"Uncle Mike, I would love some predominantly Type 1, slow twitch, aerobic muscle fibers that are more suited to endurance tasks, please." Uncle Mike is sure to be amazed ....or consider you insane.

Like every muscles in our body the pelvic floor is also home to both slow and fast twitch muscle fibers

and the latter is more suitable to powerful, fast contractions (Think orgasm...because it's exactly what an orgasm actually is. It's an involuntary, rapid contractions in the pelvic floor muscle. Science. It's now clear!) while the former is more suitable for endurance (Think postsural support and stabilization of your pelvis throughout the day).

To effectively strengthen the pelvic floor and achieve both strength as well as endurance, we must to think carefully about the training regimen we follow. Kegels in the traditional way are taught in quick, easy flashes or contractions to the pelvic floor to your maximum force of contraction. It's an excellent technique to build the quick muscles of the floor of your pelvis! But what happens to the slow fibers? An excellent way to alter the kegel exercise to target muscles with slow twitch fibers is to do the kegel for a period of 10 seconds, and then gradually increase it to 15 seconds, the next step is to see if you are able raise the intensity to 20 seconds. In all honesty, when I started my first workout my pelvic floor ached to give up within about 8 seconds. Since when.

61

It is also important to concentrate on the coordination and control of your pelvic floor. An effective way to achieve is to imagine the pelvic floor controls the elevator. Engage the pelvis as much as you can, to propel an elevator to the fifth floor. You can now ease the contracture just enough for the elevator to be on 4.

3rd floor? 2nd floor? 1st floor? Do you want to go back to 3rd floor? Then the first floor, and finally the 5th floor?

You could perform the Pelvic Floor Kegel training (let's simply label it "Intimate Weight Lifting" because the term is beginning to become more popular with me!) in your yoga mat prior to a yoga class, or when you take breaks in your child's posture to re-connect to your breathing. Also, you can do this kegel-cise on a daily basis. What's great about these exercises is that nobody will be aware that you're doing them!

Take a look! I'm in negotiations for a raise my boss.

strengthening my pelvic floor the simultaneously! "winning" means breaking up with a toxic relationship while developing a healthier connection with my body at the same time. The sequence that I typically follow approximately 1-2x per day:

10-20 quick flicks of 50% maximal contraction

1020 minutes of long contraction that holds the maximum amount of the contraction time for 10 seconds each

*Elevator games until I see my muscles becoming exhausted and require a break.

62

Important PSA: To be able to know if kegels are the best friend or enemy it is essential to have an Pelvic Health PT team to assess the muscles in your pelvic floor.

If you're suffering from excessively tense pelvic floor then the kegels you are taking in may not be exactly what you need right this moment, and you may be creating more harm than beneficial. If you're suffering from lower pelvic floor that is hypotonic and requires extra strength, teaming with an Pelvic Health practitioner who will examine your kegel-related technique is crucial.

I also want to add the importance of pelvic health.

More than just Kegels are more than. That's just the beginning of the story for you ladies and gentlemen! Are you having questions regarding pelvic health and physical therapy? Let's connect!

This chapter is very lengthy. If you've stayed with me till the very end thank for you! Your determination and perseverance is admirable and are a magnificent unicorn ordinary mortals. We thank you for your attention and investment in discovering more about your dearest person, your body.

63

In the final section, here are a few points I'm hoping you've learned: 1.Your body is amazing!

2.Kegels do not make a difference between good and good or. The way they are used could be advantageous or destructive.

3.Having an experienced PHPT in your corner could help make a huge difference.

4.And I'm sure you'll keep your pelvic floor in mind each time you have a turkey dinner at thanksgiving Dinner along with your Uncle Mike!

64

Make sure you are aware of the pelvic floor.

Chapter 7: Your Friendly Neighborhood
Pelvic Health Physical Therapist 65

The life you live is a journey of sanctity. It is about transformation and growth, discovering and transformation. always expanding your perception of the possibilities that are available and stretching your spirit and learning to look clearly and in depth, paying attention to your inner voice, and engaging in challenging challenges with courage on every step of the path.

Your path is exactly where you're supposed to be at the moment. From here, you have only one option: creating your own life's story to an epic tale of victory and healing. the strength of character, elegance, of wisdom and strength, respect, and affection.

C A R O L I N E J O Y A D A M S

66

The journey of life is one that you must take which is why you weren't intended to travel this journey by yourself! If you, or anyone that you know is going through the path of pelvic health problems and signs, be aware that you can count on specialists who are aware of your journey and are prepared to hold your arm and guide to a better future!

If they are given the chance, health issues will take away from the person you love they'll take your happiness and your feeling of belonging and your confidence in the beauty of your body, self-love and admiration, as well as some time away from people that whom you adore in this world. If you don't invest in the health of your pelvic region, along with general health and wellbeing can be too expensive.

Don't believe in the myths that because you have symptoms that are not uncommon that they are not normal. Don't believe that you're alone from your experience and must to suffer silently for a moment. Don't spend another second in this world feeling helpless in your struggles, ignored, and unrecognised.

I'd wish to introduce you an individual who could be of assistance!

67

The Pelvic Health Therapists (PHPTs) are experts in musculoskeletal health with specialized qualifications and education on pelvic health. In contrast to other healthcare professions which are trained to treat patients by piecemeal approach that focuses on assessing and treating the two or three organs or parts of the body. PHPT has a unique approach to treatment.

It is trained to look at the WHOLE individual and to manage the body holistically.

This type of evaluation and treatment is crucial! The human body isn't an instrument it's an alive, breathing very coordinated, interwoven and interdependent system.

Some people might have felt marginalized or even ignored in the health system before by an approach to medicine which does not include the complexity of the human body as well as the importance of connective tissue between the brain and body, or the interconnected nature of the human being in general.

The current system of healthcare within America United States is often quick to give prescriptions or surgeries, however it is often not able to take in the personal stories and experiences of patients or clients to determine the cause behind many issues. The PHPTs have been trained to look at things in a different way we know that you are the most important source of information about the state of your personal body. We trust in your abilities and your sense of smell, and can assist you in deciphering the messages and SOS messages that your body emits as if it's shooting flares in the dark looking for assistance!

68

PHPTs will never be on their own. We aim to become an a valuable asset and a part of your health team.

Every person needs a group that is knowledgeable and dependable to help them regardless of the path they're taking! PHPTs are a part of specialized doctors like gynecologists, sexual teachers and therapists Doulas, midwives and doulas personal trainers and counselors to offer education and support.

Utilizing the expertise of experts and being in an inter-disciplinary team is the most effective approach to ensure that people suffering from pelvic health problems receive the treatment and assistance they require. All of us are on the same team!

So What Does a Pelvic Health Evaluation Look Like?

In your first evaluation, using a PHPT complete history of your life will be taken. It will also be possible to have time and the space with your physician to share the story of your life, talk about your story, and explore your path to recovery. The clinician will ask you concerns about your physical symptoms, labor and delivery background, your preferences for movement and interests in athletics, the way your health issues affect your lifestyle, your objectives regarding your health and well-being along with co-morbidity and previous treatment.

69

A physical assessment will follow in which the PHPT will assess your movement, identify areas of weakness/compensations, test your coordination and body awareness, look for deficits in the neuromuscular system, and complete a full assessment of your pelvic floor function with your consent.

Consent is a highly respected and valued right within our area of expertise! We won't ever request you to take part in any some aspect of the evaluation that you don't want to go through.

That raises the issue of how PHPTs evaluate the muscles of the pelvic floor. ....

A pelvic health exam that is internal differs from the type you've experienced at the gynecologist's clinic. They do not employ stirrups or speculum and are intended to be totally pain-free.

During an examination that is internal on an internal exam, the PHPT uses the use of a gloved and lubricated fingers (we refer to it as"bioprobe") "bioprobe") inserted into the vagina or into the anus region to examine the three layers of pelvic floor muscle. It is possible to relax and contract your pelvic floor several times to determine the force of contracting and the coordination of muscle relaxation are examined.

You are absolutely able to be a part of a PHPT without having to undergo an internal examination However, these tests are strongly recommended since they provide your therapist with important data regarding the health the pelvic floor which is not possible to collect without.

But, as we have stated before that YOU have the control of the exam process and all of your desires will be honored!

70

After the initial evaluation has been completed, you together with the PHPT are scheduled to sit down together and talk about the results. There could be an "Ah-ha" moment in your physical health, while your doctor explains the physiological and psychological reasons that explains the various symtpoms you've experienced!

The following step of the process is to create the game plan to heal and rehabilitation. The plan is developed by the therapist and you, and will be tailored to meet the individual needs and goals of each. The Patient/Client

The Therapist Team is an effective power for good! Remember that YOU as a client are the center of the show. And just like every aspect of life the more you believe and adhere to the procedure of your PHPT more, the better the quality of your experience, and more successful your outcomes are likely to be!

After that, the fun is on! The PHPT will be in contact with all the healthcare professionals who are in your corner and, keeping your particular objectives in mind, lead your on the path in learning to appreciate and trust in your body! Exercises to enhance strength and cooridnation of the body, mindfulness and body awareness, YOGA, education using models, neruo re-education utilizing various instruments/modalities, pelvic health-specific tools, and specialized rehabilitation techniques are just some of the tools in the PHPT Toolbox that may be employed to restore your health and function throughout the process. It is essential to inform your PHPT of the changes you notice on your body or of your symptoms during the process. Communication is essential!

71

PHPTs are used in a range of different settings, from hospitals

as well as outpatient clinics. fitness centers and the convenience and comfort

Your own house.

If you're not able to make an appointment in person using a PHPT, or you are

In the event that you cannot locate a physician within your region, be aware of this

Many PHPTs offer the services of Telehealth. Go to page 78 of this guide to locate the nearest PHPT!

Be aware that it's never too late to reap the benefits of Pelvic Health Physical Therapy! If your children are five or more, you can benefit from Pelvic Health Physical Therapy!

Months or even 50 years old, or are suffering from symptoms in the last few months or over the past couple of decades, Pelvic Health Physical Therapy may be the answer!

72

The body of your precious companion in life. It's incredible and is able to treat.

Your hope is worthy and the healing.

Your voice will be heard, and will be heard.

There was no way to live life by yourself

You can take the Pelvic Health PT along with you!

73

Make sure you are aware of the pelvic floor.

A Letter

From

The author

74

I am grateful that you have joined me in this endeavor to connect the dots between science and art of yoga with regards the subject of Pelvic Health. It was my pleasure to serve as your teacher!

Thank your decision to purchase this book, and investing in yourself. The fastest way to transform the world is by changing yourself. We thank you for being participant in the evolution of the world!

This book should fill your brain of new knowledge and instilled a sense of love of your amazing, divine body and infused your soul with a desire to become the voice of The Pelvic Health Movement on and off your mat! It is your chance to help billions of people in the world (perhaps even you) that are afflicted by pelvic health issues through connecting them with information and resources (like this one!) Inviting people to use the help from an Pelvic Health PT. You can also help be an attentive listener and warm embrace to those who are willing to bravely step forward and seek assistance!

The hope-filled message and healing Pelvic Health Education and Treatment offers can transform the world! Thanks for being a part of the change that is happening in your own life and in those of your friends!

Chapter 8: What is Chronic Pelvic Pain?

The medical profession is aware that the chronic pelvic pain (CPP) isn't just one of the most common problems, but alsan extremely challenging one at that. CPP is not well understood due tthe lack of clarity regarding its cause as well as its complicated nature. The condition is often not properly managed.

In order tmanage this condition effectively it is a multidisciplinary approach necessary. Integrating and understanding every pelvic organ system vital. The neurologic, musculoskeletal and psychiatric systems should alsbe examined. There is a tendency for patients texperience other health issues, such as the bowel or bladder problem as well as sexual dysfunction, among different symptoms. Anxiety, depression and even substance abuse, can often occur.

Pain in the pelvis that is chronic which isn't caused by menstrual cycle and can last at least three months. The pain is experienced in the pelvis or beneath the belly button, and alsbehind the hips. The pain is sintense that it interferes with the normal motion that the person is experiencing. This requires either surgical or medical treatment.

In addition thaving a medical problem as a whole, persistent pelvic pain may be sign of a illness. If a doctor finds what is causing the pain, then treatment will be geared toward the condition.

Statistical Data

A chronic pelvic pain can affect around 1 in 7 women.

Research suggests that 33% of women suffer from pelvic pain during their life time.

Sixty percent of women suffering from painful pelvic issues aren't diagnosed.

There's 39% of painful pelvic aches in menopausal women, particularly those whare between 26 and 30 years old.

African-Americans have a higher prevalence of pelvic discomfort.

There isn't an organic basis for the pain that has been observed during laparoscopy, in at most 33% of instances.

30 percent of women with persistent pelvic pain underwent an operation called a Hysterectomy.

10 percent of all hysterectomies performed have been performed ttreat chronic pelvic pain.

About 20% of laparoscopies performed are due tpersistent pelvic discomfort.

Aproximately 25 percent of patients remain restless for up tthree days a month.

Approximately 60 percent of the patients don't get a diagnosis.

Causes and Symptoms of Chronic Pelvic Pain

Many conditions could result in persistent pelvic pain. A few of these issues could be caused by the urinary tract, or the bowel, instead of reproductive organs. In some women, several conditions could be the cause of their discomfort, while other women, nroot cause has been identified. Pelvic pain may develop in a variety of reasons. For added aggravation mental factors can worsen the problem. The stress of dealing with pain can't pinpoint the source of stress anyone.

The most well-known causes of the chronic pelvic pain is:

Endometriosis: When the uterus's tissue extends beyond the uterus The condition is referred tas endometriosis. It is most often present on the ovaries, fallopian tubes and on the tissue that holds the uterus as well as on the outside of the inside of the uterus. The other places where growths can occur are those of the cervix, vagina the vulva, the bowel, or the rectum. The tissue deposits function as the lining of the uterus with regard tmenstrual cycles. They become thicker, degrade and then flow out in blood, but since they're not part within the uterus they're unable tbe able texit via the vagina. They are confined tthe abdominal cavity and can result in painful cysts and adhesions. These can alslead tproblems within the bladder and intestines.

Here are some signs of endometriosis

Pelvic cramps and pain prior tand during the period

The pain can occur during or immediately after sexual contact

Pain during ovulation

Painful defecation

Urinary pain

Rectal bleeding during menstruation

Bloating in the abdomen

A lower backache

Infertility

Spotting between menstrual period

Adenomyosis Adenomyosis Adenomyosis occurs in the case of endometrial tissue that is present inside and expands tthe muscle wall that surrounds the uterus. The majority of cases occur in the last few months of child-bearing and is usually gone after menopausal changes. The condition can be discomforting and may result in pelvic discomfort. There are a few treatments that can ease the pain, however the most effective treatment for adenomyosis is surgery called hysterectomy. A majority of women suffering from adenomyosis suffer unaffected.

A few symptoms are:

Pain during menstrual period

Heavy menstrual period

Periods that last for longer than normal

Spotting between periods

A feeling of pressure or pressure sensation in the bladder or rectum

Fibroids are benign growths of the uterus which typically appear during pregnancy years. Around 3 of 4 women will experience uterine fibroids in their lives. However, the vast majority people aren't aware of it because they don't have indications. Fibroids are discovered by doctors during an exam of the pelvis or a an ultrasound scan prior tpregnancy. The fibroids can lead tdiscomfort or pressure in the pelvis as they lose blood supply, and they then begin tdeteriorate.

A few symptoms are:

Heavy menstrual periods

Hemorrhoids

Constipation

Feeling fullness or pressure within the abdomen

You may need tgtthe bathroom frequently.

Menstrual cramps

Ovarian cysts Ovarian cysts are sacs filled with fluid which develop around the an ovary. They're common, particularly when you are pregnant. Ovarian cysts are painful as they become twisted and then explodes.

The signs of ovarian cysts consist of:

Obstructive abdominal bloating or swelling

Painful defecation

Painful sex

The pain in the Pelvic area can occur before or during menstrual cycle

The pain may be from the back of your lower, or legs

Breast tenderness

Nausea and vomiting

The pelvic floor muscles. The pelvic floor is prone ttension. It occurs when pelvic floor muscles get weak, stretched or totightly. Certain pelvic floor muscles begin tlose strength at a young stage, and in other cases this happens in menopausal, pregnancy or childbirth. The muscles in the pelvic floor weaken because of a variety of factors. A few of these reasons aren't making them more active, or are overworking the muscles, including pregnancies, births and obesity. Other causes include constipation that continues for a long time or the weight of work, chronic cough injuries and older age.

The symptoms include:

Leaking urine

Feeling as if there's a fluttering in the vagina

A lower backache

Pain during sex

The difficulty of the process of defecating

The Pelvic organs can bulge out in the vagina, or extend out from the vaginal openings in extreme situations

Chronic pelvic inflammatory disorder Chronic pelvic inflammatory disorder is an infection that affects the reproductive organs of females. It is among the most dangerous consequences of STD is that it could result in permanent damage tthe ovaries, the uterus the fallopian tube, and different parts of the reproductive system. PID is a condition that occurs in the event that the cervix gets subject tan STD such as gonorrhea, or the chlamydia. The infection can spread torgans within the body.

The indicators of pelvic inflammatory disorder include:

Unique smell, texture and color of vaginal discharge

A pelvic or abdominal pain within a particular location. The pain can be more widespread for the other patients.

Missed or irregular times

Menstrual cramps that appear more severe than normal

Urinate often

Pain during urination

The pain when you ovulate

Nausea

Fever

A Tire

The lower back is a common cause of pain.

Some areas of the pelvis can hurt when you press them

Irritable bowel syndrome It is a condition which affects the colon. The condition causes stomach pain, bloating as well as constipation and diarrhea. Irritable bowel syndrome is chronic disease that requires a an ongoing management. The treatment is through a healthy life style, diet and tension.

The symptoms include:

Diarrhea

Constipation

Incontinence

Flatulence

Bloating

The relief of pain can be found in the movement of the bowel

Ovarian residual syndrome It occurs when the ovarian tissue remains after surgery tremove the fallopian tubes and both ovaries is performed. Ovarian tissue can cause intense pelvic pain, as well as a the pelvic area texpand. It could be as a result of increased usage of laparoscopic procedures which involve the surgeon operating by making twor three small incisions rather than a huge cut in the abdomen. The other factors that can increase the possibility of an incomplete removal of the ovaries include endometriosis pelvic inflammation, previous procedures for the pelvis and adhesions in the pelvis. Adhesions attach torgans and other tissues, making it hard for surgeons tdetermine and eliminate the ovaries.

A few of the signs are:

Constant, ongoing pelvic discomfort

Painful sex

Urinary pain

Painful defecation

Interstitial Cystitis - This is a persistent condition in which there's pressure in the bladder or pain in the bladder, as well as pelvic pain that can range from mild discomfort tintense painfulness. The bladder is a muscular organ which is the one that stores urine. If it's filled the bladder expands, signaling tthe brain that it's time for you tflush. For patients with interstitial cystitis, these signals can be confused. The patients feel the need tgfor a urination even though the bladder isn't completely filled.

A few of the signs are:

A need tpee often

Urinate "right now"

UTI discomfort

Painful sex

Pelvic vein congestion Alscommonly referred tas the ovarian vein reflux. It is due tthe chronic pelvic pain of 13-40% of females. It is an uncomfortable issue caused due tthe dilatation of the pelvic or ovarian veins. These veins are similar tvaricose within the pelvis.

Here are a few signs:

The pain usually begins 7 t10 days prior tmenstrual flow

Pain during sex

The pain in the Pelvic region increases while standing or sitting

The act of lying down eases discomfort

The lower back is a common cause of pain.

Aches and pains in the legs

Chronic ectopic pregnancies - A normal pregnancy occurs when the fertilized egg is transferred intthe uterus. It then joins its lining, which grows over nine months. When an ectopic pregnancy occurs, the fertilized egg remains inside the tube of fallopian tubes. In some cases, it is attached tthe Ovaries, the horns of the uterus or even tthe cervical cervix. Ectopic pregnancy requires emergency intervention.

The signs of an ectopic pregnancy include:

Light vaginal bleeding

Nausea and vomiting that causes discomfort

The lower abdomen painfulness

Sharp abdominal cramps

The neck, shoulder or the rectum

or an individual side

The weakness and dizziness can be a sign of weakness.

If the fallopian tube is ruptured, the bleeding and pain could be ssevere that it could cause fainting.

Uterus Prolapse The uterus is kept by the pelvis through a myriad of ligaments, muscles, and tissues. Birth, labor difficulties and birth can weaken the muscles. Loss of estrogen and age may lead tthe uterus falling in the canal of vaginal birth.

The signs of prolapsed uterus are as follows:

A feeling of pressure or fullness in the pelvis

A Low backache

It is a feeling that something's being released from the vagina

Pain during sex

Trouble in urinating

A difficulty in urinating

Walking is difficult.

Hernia Hernia Hernia can occur when a organ presses against an opening in the muscle tissues that hold it. It is most commonly seen in the abdominal area. In the case of the intestines could penetrate a weak point inside the abdomen wall.

For inguinal, femoral umbilical, and incisional hernias the symptoms include:

A visible swelling under the skin of your abdominal area or the groin, which could disappear when lying down

A feeling of heavyness within the abdomen which may be caused by constipation, and bloody stool.

A ache in the abdominal or groin area when bent or lifting

If you are experiencing symptoms that get worse until you are unable tsleeping patterns, causes you thave ttake time off work, and is getting impeding the routine of your day, it's the time tconsult with an expert.

Chapter 9: Diagnosing Chronic Pelvic Pain

In this chapter, I will discuss the diagnosis of chronic pelvic pain, I'll frequently refer tthe patient whis being evaluated as a patient. If you are suffering with pelvic pain and you are reading the book, of course patients refer tyou.

As per the International Pelvic Pain Society, 61 percent of women whsuffer from persistent pelvic pain dnot know what is causing their condition. When the diagnosis is correct the relief of pain is likely. There are experts you can assist you in determining what is causing your discomfort, and then suggest what you could dtake talleviate it.

Most often, patients see with a gynecologist if they suffer from an ongoing pelvic discomfort. Gynecologists may recommend the patient ta different specialist for treatment, like:

Urologist- If, such as, symptoms and pelvic examination suggest the presence of interstitial cystitis, there's the tests that a doctor can perform. A cystoscopy may be performed for a look at the bladder for bleeding and ulcers. Also, he can perform tests for potassium sensitivity in which he fills the bladder up with a potassium solution followed by water. Patients with cystitis interstitial feel the pain and have a strong urge tgfor a urination with potassium, rather instead of water.

Gastroenterologist: The gastroenterologist specialises in digestive issues. Patients may have consult one due tthe fact that the condition known as irritable bowel syndrome (IBS) is one of the main causes of pelvic discomfort. It is often not the primary cause however there are occasions where it is accompanied by other reasons.

Pain Specialists - Pain specialists are doctors of anesthesia whhave been specially are trained tmanage pain. They are able tcomplement treatment offered by a general practitioner or Gynecologists. Specialists in pain are required for the proper testing of nerve blocks and the application of TENS transcutaneous electrical nerve stimulation (TENS) devices, or for medication control.

Physical Therapist - A physical therapist may develop an exercises program as well as relaxation methods which can help strengthen pelvic floor muscles and reduce the pain, and reduce anxiety and stress.

Psychiatrist/Psychologist - A psychiatrist and psychologist can help even if the physical source of pelvic pain has been identified. The mind plays an important part in the perception of discomfort. Stress, depression and anxiety are alsable tmake discomfort appear tbe more severe.

Before visiting the Gynecologist or primary care doctor Dthe following as part of your pre-treatment:

Record all modifications you see on your body. This includes ones you believe may not be related tthe cause of your discomfort.

Record all latest changes that have occurred in your life. A few of them may create stress in you that you aren't aware of.

Create a list of your medications that you're using.

Try ttake your companion along. Your companion could help provide more accurate information tthe doctor if you don't remember some thing.

Write down everything you would like your doctor tsay for example:

What might be the reasons for your suffering?

Which tests are you required ttake and how can you be prepared for these tests?

What are available treatment options for you?

What is the period of treatment?

How long will it take texperience relief from discomfort?

Dyou have reading material you can read thelp educate yourself about the condition?

Doctors will ask questions. These include:

When did you begin experiencing sensation? What is the frequency you experience it? Does the pain change over the course of time? How much is the hurt? How long will it last?

What is the location where area of pain? Dyou experience the pain elsewhere or is it the same spot?

Dyou feel discomfort while you urinate? Are you able tfeel discomfort when you urinate?

Dyou think your menstrual cycle could cause discomfort?

Dyou have anything you can could dtlessen the discomfort? Dyou have any habits which could make your pain even more painful?

Are you able tfunction at a comfortable level despite discomfort?

If yes, have you received treatment ttreat urinary tract infections or vaginal infections?

Are you a patient of the procedure for your pelvis?

Dyou remember being pregnant?

If you have been sexually or physically abused?

Have you felt depressed?

What therapies have you already tried?

*The doctor will perform a pelvic exam. He will then:

Check out how you stand and sit.

You can press on different locations throughout your pelvic and abdominal area and ask yourself tfeel pain in the area you are feeling.

Request that you tighten and loosen the pelvic muscles.

You can feel inside the uterus, vagina and rectum tdiscover something that is unusual.

In some cases, a pelvic check might be enough tdetermine the issue or a part of it at the very least. The doctor could request test results such as transvaginal ultrasonography as well as an CT scan or MRI scan of your pelvis and abdomen for an even more comprehensive image.

Finding the root of pelvic pain can be easy. There are women whdon't have the exact diagnosis for the pain. This doesn't mean that the discomfort isn't there and cannot be addressed.

A thorough history of the patient is crucial tdetermine an accurate diagnosis and a suitable treatment program. A consultation with other specialists is required in the event of connected diseases. A thorough review of digestive, gastro-intestinal, urologic and neuro-psychiatric system will assist tdetermine the diagnosis.

History

In determining the history of a patient Pay attention tdetails of the way in which pain is described.

Ask the patient tidentify the precise location that where she is experiencing pain. Take a photfor her tpinpoint the location of the area of pain.

Ask the patient about what conditions or events caused the pain in the first place and alswhat triggers pain. Answers tthese questions will allow you tdetermine the possibility of other problems. If, for instance, the discomfort is caused by the posture of a person and gets worse towards the final hours of the day, it could be due tthe pelvic constriction syndrome. In the event, on contrary, it is due in sexuality, then the woman could suffer from endometriosis.

If the patient is unsure, ask trest if it helps ease the discomfort. If the answer is yes, it could mean that the issue is of muscular or skeletal origin.

Ask your patient twrite down the sensation. Are you feeling it as if it is the sensation of crushing? Pressing? Penetrating?

Ask patient whether the pain has increased or seems tget worse.

Request the patient trate their intensity of the pain with the 10-point scale.

The history of the patient should be specific tvarious medical techniques.

Gynecologic as well as obstetric

A lot of bleeding may result from uterine issues.

A previous operation could have caused pelvic adhesions.

Multiple partners sexually can result in pelvic inflammatory.

Patients suffering from cervical stenosis might be suffering from chronic cervical infections, or may be treated by cryosurgery or endometrial removal.

Adenomyosis can cause severe pelvic pain, dysmenorrhea and endometriosis and depression. those with fibroids.

Musculoskeletal

Vaginal delivery which leads ttears can create pelvic floor stress problem.

Urologic

Assess your urological system for the purpose of ruling out cystitis interstitial. Although there may be pain with interstitial cystitis it's distinct from pelvic pain as the latter is characterised by the frequency of urine and the urgency.

Gastrointestinal

Deflecting sigmoid adhesions can be prevalent for patients suffering from chronic pelvic pain as well as being related tGI signs.

Neurologic

It is common among Pudendal Neurolgia sufferers.

Psychological

Psychosexual or psychosocial past is necessary in cases where the pain does not appear thave an organic the source. Assess anxiety disorders, depression and sexual or physical addiction, abuse of drugs or marital issues, as well as sexual issues

Abuse of sexual nature at a young age can be linked tpainful pelvic issues.

Physical Examination and Laboratory Studies

A thorough and comprehensive physical examination is crucial tmaking a diagnosis as well as an suitable treatment program. Relax the patient because some exams can be a bit difficult.

Obstetric-gynecologic examination can be long. It can be difficult for the patient. They can be performed in a variety of postures, including standing, supine, sitting as well as lithotomy position. A supine posture is where the hips and knees fully extend while the legs are separated and elevated, while the feet rest on straps.

The Lithotomy exam consists of the following:

Examining the external Genitalia.

Tests and evaluation of sensory sensation of trigger points, where a cotton-tipped, swab can be utilized for accurate sensory and tender-point assessment of the cervical os, vaginal cuff as well as the paracervical and cervical region.

A single-digit evaluation of the pubic arch, the coccyx, cervical, uterus and urethral.

Colposcopic assessment of the vestibule and vulva.

Examen of the speculum, pelvic and vaginal muscles.

Bimanual pelvic examination.

Rectovaginal Examination.

A thorough examination of the different systems, if is required.

Evaluation of posture and gait

Spine examination

Sensory exam

Motor test

The Beatty maneuver, which involves it is performed by abducting the knee in opposition tresistance is done and the patient is reported thave discomfort.

Obturator sign for testing tdetermine if there is a problem with the fascia or obturator muscles.

Straight-leg raise test tcheck for a possible herniated disc.

or Psoas indication where the hip's flexion against resistance occurs. If you feel pain or discomfort the possibility is that there's problems with the psoas muscle or fascia.

Abduction Flexion and the external rotation test as part of the hip test.

The transvaginal ultrasound scan can assist in the screening and assessment of Adnexal tumors.

Transvaginal scans and Magnetic radiography (MRI) can be useful tdiagnose Adenomyosis.

The use of urological procedures like urinalysis or urine culture are recommended. They are a low-cost laboratory procedure which should be carried out when needed. If there is a sign of hematuria it is possible thave the patient assessed using urine cytology cystourethroscopy, and an intravenous Pyelography. If malignancy is suspected doctors may request an urological cytology particularly when the patient is smoking.

CBC counts provide non-specific results however the results could be indicative of inflammation or an infection. In some cases, it could be a sign of malignancy.

A screening for a serum drug is recommended when street or prescription drugs are being used.

Testing for the presence of sexually transmitted diseases includes cervical cultures or Smears, Syphilis serology tests, hepatitis B screening, the chlamydial polymerase chain reactions and HIV screening.

Vaginal culture and vaginal wet preparations and vaginal pH can be used tdetermine particular infections.

The results of hormonal tests are likely beneficial if it is believed that ovarian remnant syndrome tbe a cause for pelvic discomfort.

The test for thyroid-stimulating hormones can be used tdetect hypothyroidism when a patient is with depression-related symptoms.

Imaging StudiesUltrasonography is an uninvasive method of diagnosis which is beneficial tthe majority of patients whsuffer from persistent pelvic pain. It helps tdetermine pelvic cysts, or pelvic masses as well as their source as well as pelvic varicosities, hernias and pelvic varico.

CT scanning can be useful when patients have pelvic masses. It can alsassist in distinguishing an ovarian mass from an uterine mass. CT scanning can be more costly than sonography.

Magnetic Resonance Imaging (MRI) is a non-invasive device which can give superior structural data without radiation-related harm. Intravenous contrast may be utilized in cases of inflammation, infection, or malignancy is suspected.

Plain film radiography can prove useful for cancers, injuries, fractures as well as other structural anomalies. Abdominal radiographs are a way tidentify intestinal obstruction as well as pelvic inflammation.

Hysterosalpingography is useful in patients with infiltrative endometriosis of the uterosacral ligaments. The test can alsbe useful for cases that suggest endometrial polyps Asherman syndrome, and adenomyosis.

Barium enema radiography colonoscopy, the upper GI series, and anorectal manometry are utilized tassess GI the underlying cause of chronic pain.

Vaginal ultrasound is a valuable tool for patients whmay have constriction of the pelvis syndrome.

The use of cystourethrography tdetect cysts is beneficial when patients are suspect of having cystitis interstitial.

Diagnostic Considerations

It is crucial tbe open when evaluating anyone whis suffering from constant painful pelvic pain. People suffering from chronic pelvic pain might appear exaggerated, and the complaints they are complaining about may appear tbe unfounded, but it is imperative that they are treated with respect.

Review your history thoroughly in order tprevent repeating the same invasive and costly procedure. Talk tother experts before taking a decision about aggressive or in-depth management.

You should be extra vigilant when treating patients whexhibit the following:

A history of sexual and physical abuse

Marriage, family, or sexual issues

Drug abuse or dependence

Insufficient response tcorrect treatment

Failure tcomply with previous treatment

A rare, unexpected reaction in response tspecific treatment prior

The behavior is considered tbe anti-social, such as the absconding of work, school or other responsibilities in social settings

Severe depression

Very severe anxiety

Pain that is tosevere

Frequent changes tthe health care provider

Take extra care when taking care of patients whare expecting.

Initial pain management needs tbe restricted tnon-pharmacologic methods including rest, reassurance and cold or hot applications as well as stretching, position exercises ultrasound therapy, massage TENS, relaxation therapy, and biofeedback. If the pain doesn't respond medications, they can be prescribed with care.

It is possible tallow medication however it must be restricted tonly when absolutely necessary.

Acetaminophen as well as codeine could be taken during the pregnancy.

Nonsteroidal anti-inflammatory medications like ibuprofen or aspirin should be considered for the first trimester, but only. Following the first trimester, these medications can cause bleeding in the fetus or maternal artery.

Chapter 10: Treating Chronic Pelvic Pain

If your doctor is capable of identifying a specific reason for the discomfort, your treatment will be focused on removing the source. In the event, on the other side, your doctor could not pinpoint the root of the problem, treatment will be focused on pain relief.

It is possible tcomplicate treatment if patients have multiple health issues. The patient will require specialized care as well as physical and mental therapy too. The purpose of treatment should be realistic. The focus should be on returning the patient's capacity tbe functional, enhance the quality of life, and avoid any relapses of the symptoms.

Medications

Doctors may prescribe medicines ttreat or lessen the severity of symptoms.

Initial, a few available over-the-counter medications could be sufficient tease the discomfort. These include:

Paracetamol

Ibuprofen

Aspirin

Naproxen

If the results are not satisfactory In the event of a negative outcome, prescription medication might be prescribed.

Antibiotics: Antibiotics can be prescribed by a doctor if he believes there is an infection tbe the reason for pain.

Antidepressants are antidepressants that may help with chronic pain-related disorders. Tricyclic antidepressants can relieve pain and can help people that aren't necessarily depressed.

Treatment for hormones Birth control pills as well as other hormone-based medications can help alleviate symptoms when pelvic pain is a result of the menstrual cycle.

Therapies

Certain treatments or procedures could constitute included in the treatment program ttreat pelvic pain that is chronic.

Triggerpoint injections An injection of medication that numbs the location where pain occurs might be suggested if the particular point is identified. The medicine used is typically a local anesthetic with a long-acting effect which can reduce the pain and relieve discomfort.

Physical therapy - - Cold or hot compression on the abdomen as well as stretching exercises and massages can help relieve persistent pelvic pain. Workouts that target strengthening of the muscles of the pelvic floor may be suggested. These and other strategies for coping could be developed by the physical therapist. The therapist can alspinpoint certain areas of pain by using TENS, or transcutaneous electric neural stimulation (TENS). It can aid in identifying regions where muscles are tight.

*Spinal cord stimulation A device will be inserted tblock neural pathways that connect that connect tthe brain. The brain won't get pain signals. It could be useful based on the cause of pelvic pain.

Psycho-physiological Therapy

Sometimes, pain may be connected with anxiety, depression or any other personal issue. Assistance with psychotherapy can be an crucial tthe treatment program. Psycho-physiological treatment includes:

Reassurance

Counseling

Relaxation therapy

Program for stress management

Biofeedback techniques

Biofeedback in conjunction with medicine has been proven useful for some patients.

Surgery

The use of minimally-invasive methods can provide relief from pain. The most common are:

The injection of trigger points is most often used tlocalize trigger points.

Blocks of peripheral nerves using local anesthetics and steroids.

Nueroablation of specific nerves may be done by using various methods, such as:

Thermocoagulation, the process of making use of electrical currents of high frequency tcause the destruction of tissue in a specific area.

Cryoablation, the usage of extreme cold in order tresult in the destruction of localized tissues.

The injection of chemicals

A morphine injection pump intrathecal can be employed for the right patients.

The stimulation of the sacral nerve could help in the management of pelvic pain syndromes that are resistant ttherapy.

Surgery is a possibility when minimally-invasive methods aren't successful. They include:

Presacral Neurocissectomy. This surgery will stop the nerves from traveling tthe infected uterus. It is regarded as the most effective method trelieve the pain of endometriosis.

*Parcervical denervation procedure is performed ttransect the uterosacral ligaments and is used primarily for relief from dysmenorrhea. This procedure is performed either via laparoscopic or vaginally.

Excision of the Uterovaginal Ganglion This is a procedure that is the removal of the hypogastric plexus in the lower part.

Laparoscopic surgery Laparoscopic surgery allows removal of adhesions, or the endometrial tissue that causes the endometriosis. Laparoscopes are inserted inttiny incisions around the navel. A second device that removes the adhesion is introduced through several small cuts.

Hysterectomy: In rare instances, a doctor might advise elimination of the uterus or the ovaries. The removal of the ovaries strips endometriosis from estrogen, and stops its development. The procedure could be a viable option for pelvic pain patients beyond the age of childbearing.

Inpatient Care

It is not necessary for patients with chronic pelvic pain. The need for it could be contingent on the degree of invasiveness in the treatment program tcontrol pain and the seriousness of the issue.

Home Remedies

What's sbad about pelvic pain is that it may cause disruption tyour daily life. It can make sleeping difficult, as well as completing your daily routine isn't as simple. There is a chance that you'll be working when your discomfort is just todifficult tmanage. The stress of this disruption can be stressful, and can aggravate the discomfort. You can try these quick solutions at home talleviate pain

Use the heating pad hot water bottle, a heating pad or warm compresses on your lower back. The heat increases blood flow, and it can relieve discomfort.

Relax in a hot bath.

If you are suffering from back pain, lay down, and then place a pillow underneath the knees, allowing you tlift the legs. While lying sideways and bringing your knees up tthe chest.

Regular exercise is a great way tincrease the flow of blood, boost endorphins and decrease the pain.

Try sexual activities that could ease backache and cramps.

Alternative Medicine

Alternative therapies could help reduce discomfort. Based on the patient's medical history or situation as well as test results the physician will determine the potential for alternative therapies taid in relieving the symptoms. The most common alternative therapies include:

Relaxation techniques: Deep breathing, as well as specific exercises tstretch the pelvic area can reduce discomfort.

Acupuncture - Endorphins(alsknown as your body's own natural painkiller release during Acupuncture treatment. Acupuncture is considered tbe as safe, but its efficacy in the treatment of pelvic pain has yet tbe proved.

Complications

Like many other chronic pains problems, pelvic pain chronically can lead tlong-lasting pain. Additionally, it can cause issues with family and marital relationships as well as loss of work or disabilities. Treatment for lifelong or ongoing may be a cause of negative medical reactions.

Chapter 11: Preventing Chronic Pelvic Pain

In the case of preventative treatment for chronic pelvic pain Early diagnosis and treatment can prevent it from becoming persistent. Since persistent pelvic pain is result of a myriad of ailments the best way tprevent it is by preventing the condition which causes it.

Condition: Pelvic Inflammatory Disease

One of the main causes of persistent pelvic pain is the pelvic inflammatory disorder. Engaging in safe sexual activity is the most effective method treduce the possibility of pelvic inflammation illness.

Practice Safe Sex

Sexually transmitted diseases (STIs) are transmitted through sexual contact through the oral cavity, the genitals or the rectum. Pregnant women can transfer it ther child prior or after delivery. The majority of sexually transmitted diseases can be eliminated, however some can't be, such as HIV as well as genital herpes. HPV (human the papillomavirus) which may cause sexual bleeding.

Individuals wharen't aware that they have contracted the disease can pass their illness tpartners. Make sure twear a protective device each time you engage in sexual activity until you're sure that neither of you are at risk.

If you're engaged, you must agree with your spouse that you'll both be monogamous. For your protection and that of your partner, your self further, you should have each of you checked for STIs.

The best method tprevent infecting yourself is tavoid any contact with sexual nature, even oral sexual contact.

Get acquainted with your partner thoroughly before engaging in any sexual relationship.

Ask your friend whthe most number of times he/she's been sexually involved with.

Did she/he have sex without condoms?

Did she/he have sexual sex that was not protected?

Have they had multiple sexual partners at one moment?

Is she/he injecting illegal substances or has had sexual sex without someone whhas?

Have they had an unprotected affair with prostitutes?

Did she/he test for HIV? What results have they returned?

Have they ever suffered from an STI? Have they been cured of it?

Be aware of signs and symptoms of STIs that include strange discharges, sores or growing or redness of the genital areas or pain during urination.

Apply a water-based oil tstop tears from the skin when there's insufficient lubrication for sexual activity. The vagina's tiny tears or rectum allow bacteria or viruses tpenetrate.

Don't take more than one sex with a partner at the same time.

Make sure tuse a condom each time.

Beware of douching as it may alter the natural balance of organisms within the vagina.

Dnot engage in sexual relations If you're affected.

Condition: Weak Musculoskeletal System

Chronic pelvic pain could be a result of muscular or skeletal issues. In order tbuild strength in the pelvic area, and alstsafeguard the area There are exercises are able thelp build and strengthen the muscles that surround the area.

Exercise

Pelvic Tilt The exercise will strengthen your lower abdominal muscles as well as the pelvic muscles.

What tdo:

1. Relax lying on the ground with your legs bent with arms at your side.

2. Engage the abdominal muscles of your lower back towards the spine. Hold for

five seconds. Take a pause before returning tthe original position.

3. Repeat the process 10-20 times.

Take note that this exercise is designed tnaturally tilt your pelvis upwards when done properly. Dnot engage gluteus or thighs while doing the exercise.

Reverse Crunch This workout is a great way tstrengthen the lower and upper abdominal muscles.

What tdo:

1. Lying on your back, you should be lying on the ground with your hips bent sthat the upper legs are parallel with the ground. The knees should bend at 90 degrees while the lower leg is in line with the floor. Maintain arms parallel teach other on the floor tprovide support.

2. The lower abs are contracted intthe spine, and then lift your hips above the flooring. Then, stop at the top of the exercise and then come back tthe starting position.

3. Perform twsets of 10-12 repetitions.

Bicycle Maneuver

The steps ttake:

1. Lay on your back lying on the ground with your feet between 10 and 12 inches from the flooring. Place your arms across the chest. This is the position tstart.

2. The right leg should be brought and the knee toward the chest, keeping the left leg straight.

3. Da semi-crunch motion by rotating your torsa bit and then bring your left elbow until it is in line with the knee

when it reaches the chest. Pause briefly before returning tyour starting place.

4. Repeat the movement by alternating the left and the right elbow until you have completed one rep.

5. Perform 25-50 repetitions.

Stretch Supine Frog This workout stretches the inside legs by pulling them back and a slackening of the hips. The buttocks are alsengaged as the frog's position is held.

What tdo:

1. Lay on the floor on your back and spread your arms extended toward the sides.

2. Begin by bringing the soles of your feet in a slack position with knees pointed out, similar tarms.

3. Letting your knees stretch and relax, allow them thang while you feel your glutes and thighs stretch.

4. In order tincrease the stretching, bring your heels tyour groin.

5. Keep the posture until you find your body relaxed and comfortable.

Supine hip rotation - This workout stretches and opens the buttocks and the hip muscles deep. The pelvis is alspositioned relative tthe spinal. For this workout the person should sit on a wall.

The steps tfollow:

1. Place your body on the floor, with both feet against the wall, with your legs in a feet approximately hip-width from each other.

2. Flex your hips and legs t90 degrees, then spread your arms on the sides.

3. The left leg is crossed across the knee of your right, ensuring that your hips don't move while doing this.

4. The left knee should be pushed towards the wall using only the left hip muscles, not the hands.

5. Maintain the pose until you are comfortable and take deep breaths intthe stretch.

6. Be careful not tover-stretch your muscles or you will trigger the reflex tstretch.

7. Take everything you can from the other side.

Supine Adduction/Abduction exercise is comprised of twpelvic exercises which help strengthen the muscles surrounding the hip joint. The equipment required is a flexible strap or belt, as well as an exercise pad or block. The hip abduction process is the movement of the legs away from center in the human body. Adduction of the hips is the movement of legs towards the body's center. The exercise targets the both adduction and abduction.

The steps tfollow:

1. Lay on your back, while keeping your knees bent with your feet resting on the floor. Your knees, hips and feet must be straight in a in a straight line.

2. Put the cushion in between your ankles, and then wrap the straps around your legs just above the knees.

3. Place your arms on the sides, palms raised.

4. Then, press the ankles teach other and simultaneously pushing the knees forward.

5. Then release the pattern three times with 10 repetitions per set. Don't turn the soles of your feet toward the cushion, or raise your heels as you push.

6. The next time you exercise, put the cushion between knees, and wrap put the strap on the ankles, keeping the feet hip width teach other.

7. Try the opposite exercise tthe earlier exercise, pulling your knees towards each other and pulling the ankles away.

8. Make sure you squeeze your knees and press against the strap using your ankles.

9. Release, and repeat the next three sets, 10 times.

Condition: Weak Pelvic Floor Muscles

The pelvic floor muscles is a different reason for chronic pelvic discomfort.

There are exercises are a good way tincrease the strength and endurance of the pelvic floor. In order tlocate the muscles in your pelvic floor, visualize the muscles that you contract while you hold your bladder. Then, you can train these muscles up and inward instead of going down and out.

Exercise

Madonna

What tdo:

1. With a yoga mat rest your back on your heels then spread the knees out mat-wide and place your hands on your back. Point them towards the sky.

2. Maintain the abs in a state of engagement and the spine is neutral. Bring the hips upwards. Maintain your chin in a straight line toward your chest, or let your head drop tthe side.

3. DKegel exercises and tighten your muscles like you were holding your pee while your hips are elevated.

4. The muscles should be engaged slowly. remain for five seconds before you let them gat a slow pace.

5. Lower the hips, then repeat the 10 times.

Pelvic Lift

The steps ttake:

1. Straighten your legs in front and spread them a bit wider in front of the hips.

2. Bring your hips upwards and then keep your chin in a tucked position towards your chest, or let your head drop tthe side.

3. Perform Kegel exercises as your hips are elevated.

4. Engage the pelvic muscles ta single rep, and before releasing.

5. Reduce the hips tthe floor and repeat the 10 times.

Shiva

The steps ttake:

1. Relax on your back with your hands resting behind your body and your feet resting on the flooring. The knees should align with your toes.

2. Make sure that your abs, ribcage and glutes engaged while you elevate your hips until the base the shoulder blades. In this elevated position, increase the speed of your pulse and then down.

3. Perform Kegel exercises as your hips are raised.

4. The muscles are contracted three tfour times and breathe slowly. Relax and take an inhalation. Repeat.

5. Lower the hips and repeat 10 times.

Good Nutrition

There is a possibility that the food you consume can tprevent chronic discomfort. Studies suggest that there's an association between diet and the way our bodies deal with discomfort.

Inflammation is a key factor in chronic discomfort. It's the body's normal response tinjury that can cause chronic suffering. There are proteins within our body that are known as "cytokines" that interacts with the your immune system. It regulates the body's responses tdiseases and infections. The body alsdevelops susceptibility tdiscomfort. Through a healthy diet we can lower the levels of these pro-inflammatory cells known as cytokines. Nutritional health is crucial ttreat chronic suffering.

There are just twmain guidelines tadhere tregarding nutrition and managing pain. The first one concerns the rate at which our bodies absorb sugar. The more slowly the body process sugar, the more efficiently it will be able tdeal with inflammation. A major study has found that inflammation can be high among women wheat foods that have a the highest glycemic score. This study alsshows the foods with higher levels on the glycemic scale have a higher risk of causing inflammation and discomfort. These aren't a great option for managing pain.

The other rule concerns how tmanage consumption of omega-3 fats with omega-6 acid fatty acids. Essential fatty acids cannot be made by our body, they come by eating. In terms of the management of pain, we need tattain a healthy balance between omega-3 and omega-6 acid fatty acids. There are only a handful of sources of omega-3 fats. In addition tthe fats found in fish that are cold-water, we are able tget them only from flaxseeds, walnuts, avocadolive oil and enhanced eggs. Omega-6 fatty acids in contrast, can be readily available in our food. They can be found in seeds, nuts, and oils they produce. The majority of the animals consumed are fed by grains and syou receive omega-6 from grains too. The vast difference between omega-3 and omega-6 can be attributed tthe extremely low amount of the former as well as the high amount of omega-6. This is an issue with regard tinflammation as omega-3 and omega-6 both have distinct impacts when it comes tthe process. Omega-6 can cause more inflammation, while omega-3 reduces inflammation. In summary these important things tconsider regarding eating right and managing pain.

Tdecrease the amount of celluloid cytokines that are present in our bodies limit the consumption of food items with the highest glucose load. They are the foods that trigger sudden rises and decreases in the levels of insulin. These include:

White bread

Potatoes

Ceral

Rice

White flour

Foods processed

Eat more food items which are rich in omega-3 acid. They're beneficial for reducing inflammation. They include:

Fish that is cold water (salmon herring, sardines mackerel, herring)

Walnuts

Leafy green vegetables

Ground flax seed flax oil

Reduce consumption of food items that are high in omega-6 and trans fats. A few of them are:

Read about meats

Dairy items

Hydrogenated oils that are partially hydrogenated

Corn, cottonseed peanuts, grapeseeds Soy, Safflower, sunflower oils

Foods that have a long shelf-life, like chips or crackers

Eat food items that are abundant in antioxidants like:

Orange, yellow and red veggies (peppers and carrots)

Allium veggies (onions and garlic)

Dark greens (spinach and romaine lettuce)

Citrus fruits

Green and black teas

Make sure tuse spices with anti-inflammatory ingredients such as

Ginger

Nutmeg

Rosemary

or Oregano

Turmeric

Cayenne

Clove

Use herbal remedies that possess anti-inflammatory properties like:

Feverfew

Willow bark

Boswellia

Limit the consumption of processed foods.

Limit intake of hydrogenated fats

Avoid consumption of animal products as well as dairy products.

Consume more vegetables and fruits that are freshly picked since they're great foods that can help reduce inflammation.

You should aim teat around 30 grams a every day.

Check the labels on food products tensure there's not excessive chemical additives.

www.ingramcontent.com/pod-product-compliance
Lightning Source LLC
Chambersburg PA
CBHW051727020426
42333CB00014B/1192